# Pcos Diet Cookbook 2023:

## Healthy And Nourished Recipes

Dr. Louvenia W. Williamson

# Table of Content

# Introduction to the PCOS Diet Cookbook

The PCOS Diet Cookbook is a complete guide to controlling Polycystic Ovary Syndrome (PCOS) via clean and nutritious food. This cookbook contains tasty, nutrient-dense dishes free from processed foods, sugar, and other elements that might increase PCOS symptoms.

With chapters on breakfast, snacks and appetizers, main dishes, side dishes, and desserts, this cookbook provides a broad selection of delectable and fulfilling meals that are simple to make and will leave you feeling invigorated. Also, this book contains recommendations for switching to the PCOS diet, food planning, and adhering to the diet long-term. Whether you're a seasoned PCOS dieter or new to the lifestyle, The PCOS Diet Cookbook is a crucial resource for anybody wishing to better their health and control their symptoms via tasty, therapeutic meals.

# CHAPTER ONE

1.0 What is PCOS?

PCOS stands for Polycystic Ovary Syndrome.

PCOS is a syndrome in which women have an imbalance of reproductive hormones; frequently, the ovaries generate an excess of the male hormone, testosterone, and a deficiency of the female hormone, estrogen. Consequently, the body doesn't go through regular ovulation, so the eggs not adequately released each month typically enlarge and cluster around the ovaries, producing cysts.

Since the body's estrogen receptors don't operate correctly, its entire metabolic system may be thrown off, disrupting everything from how it processes insulin to the healthy bacteria in the gut microbiome. A Gynecologist's Lifeline to Naturally Recover Your Rhythms, Hormones, and Happiness.

According to the U.S. Department of Health and Human Services, the illness officially affects 10 percent of American women (and frequently their fertility). Still, physicians estimate it's more like 25 percent since many instances go undetected or rejected.

## 1.1 SYMPTOMS OF PCOS

Polycystic ovarian syndrome (PCOS) is a hormonal condition that affects women of reproductive age.

The symptoms of PCOS might vary from person to person. However, frequent indications and symptoms include:

**1. Irregular periods:** PCOS may cause irregular, infrequent, or missing periods.

**2. Excess androgen:** High amounts of androgen (male hormones) may promote excess hair growth on the face, chest, stomach, back, and buttocks. Androgen may also induce acne and male pattern baldness.

**3. Polycystic ovaries:** The ovaries may grow larger and contain numerous tiny cysts, which may cause pelvic pain and discomfort.

**4. Weight gain:** Women with PCOS may have difficulties reducing weight or may gain weight rapidly.

**5. Insulin resistance:** Some women with PCOS have insulin resistance, which may lead to elevated blood sugar levels and an increased risk of developing type 2 diabetes.

**6. Emotional changes:** PCOS may induce mood swings, despair, and anxiety.

**7. Infertility:** PCOS is a primary reason for infertility in women.

It's crucial to note that not all women with PCOS may have all of these symptoms, and other people may not experience any symptoms at all. If you feel you may have PCOS, it's crucial to go to your healthcare professional for diagnosis and treatment.

# 1.2 How nutrition might affect PCOS symptoms

Polycystic ovarian syndrome (PCOS) is a hormonal condition that affects women of reproductive age. It is characterized by numerous cysts in the ovaries, irregular menstrual cycles, high levels of androgens (male hormones), and insulin resistance.

Food may play a crucial role in controlling PCOS symptoms. In this response, we will cover how nutrition affects PCOS symptoms.

**Insulin Resistance:** Women with PCOS commonly have insulin resistance, which means their systems cannot utilize insulin efficiently, leading to greater insulin levels in circulation. This may promote weight gain, type 2 diabetes, and increased production of androgens.

Consuming a diet heavy in refined carbs and sugar might cause insulin resistance. Certain foods promote a jump in blood sugar levels, leading to an increase in insulin production. On the other hand, a low-glycemic index diet, which contains whole grains, fruits, vegetables, and lean protein sources, may enhance insulin sensitivity and lower insulin levels.

**Weight Management:** Women with PCOS are at an increased risk of acquiring obese, which may worsen PCOS symptoms. Reducing weight may help improve insulin resistance, regulate menstrual cycles, and lower testosterone levels. A balanced and nutritious diet that contains a range of foods, such as lean protein, healthy fats, and complex carbs, may help control weight and enhance overall health.

**Inflammation:** Inflammation may increase PCOS symptoms and contribute to the development of insulin resistance. Eating meals heavy in saturated and trans fats, such as red meat, processed foods, and fried foods, may promote inflammation. Conversely, ingesting foods high in antioxidants like fruits, vegetables, whole grains, and nuts may help decrease inflammation.

**Hormone Balance:** PCOS is a hormone condition, and food may alter hormone balance. Eating foods strong in phytoestrogens, such as soy-based meals, may help regulate hormone levels. Moreover, ingesting foods abundant in fiber, such as fruits, vegetables, and whole grains, may help control estrogen levels.

**Gut Health:** Gut microbiota plays a crucial role in general health, and there is rising evidence that it may play a role in PCOS. Eating a diet rich in fiber, prebiotics, and probiotics may improve gut health and decrease inflammation, which can help control PCOS symptoms.

In conclusion, nutrition may have a substantial influence on PCOS symptoms. Eating a balanced and nutritious diet that is low in refined carbohydrates, sugar, and saturated and trans fats and high in whole grains, fruits, vegetables, lean protein, and healthy fats can help manage PCOS symptoms by reducing insulin resistance, controlling weight, reducing inflammation, balancing hormones, and improving gut health. It is always a good idea to visit a healthcare practitioner or a qualified dietitian for individualized guidance on treating PCOS symptoms via nutrition.

## 1.3 Advantages of adopting the PCOS diet

Polycystic Ovary Syndrome (PCOS) is a hormonal condition that affects many women of reproductive age. It is characterized by excessive androgens (male hormones) and insulin resistance, which may lead to irregular menstruation periods, ovarian cysts, weight gain, acne, and increased hair growth. Although there is no treatment for PCOS, adopting a PCOS diet may help control symptoms and improve overall health.

These are some of the advantages of adopting a PCOS diet:

**Helps manage insulin levels:** Insulin resistance is a significant aspect of PCOS, which may cause high blood sugar levels, weight gain, and type 2 diabetes. A PCOS diet may help manage insulin levels by decreasing the intake of refined carbs and sweets and increasing the consumption of complex carbohydrates, fiber, and protein. This may enhance insulin sensitivity and minimize the chance of acquiring type 2 diabetes.

**Reduces inflammation:** Inflammation contributes to many chronic diseases, including PCOS. A PCOS diet emphasizes whole, nutrient-dense foods, such as fruits, vegetables, whole grains, and healthy fats, which are rich in antioxidants and anti-inflammatory compounds. This can reduce inflammation in the body, improve overall health, and manage PCOS symptoms.

**Promotes weight loss:** Excess weight and obesity are standard in women with PCOS and can worsen symptoms. A PCOS diet may assist in promoting weight reduction by decreasing the intake of processed and high-calorie meals and boosting the consumption of nutrient-dense whole foods that promote fullness and satisfaction. Moreover, some research shows that a low-carbohydrate diet may benefit weight reduction in women with PCOS.

**Improves menstrual periods:** Irregular menstrual cycles are characteristic of PCOS, which may contribute to problems conceiving and other reproductive concerns.

A PCOS diet may help regulate menstrual periods by boosting insulin sensitivity and lowering inflammation. Also, some studies show that a diet high in omega-3 fatty acids may enhance menstrual cycle regularity in individuals with PCOS.

**Reduces androgen levels:** Excessive levels of androgens, such as testosterone, are a typical characteristic of PCOS and may cause acne, excess hair growth, and other symptoms. A PCOS diet may help lower androgen levels by increasing weight reduction, enhancing insulin sensitivity, and decreasing inflammation.

**Increases fertility:** PCOS is a common cause of infertility in women, and adopting a PCOS diet may enhance fertility by controlling menstrual cycles, lowering androgen levels, and increasing weight reduction. Also, a diet high in minerals, such as folate, zinc, and iron, may improve fertility in women with PCOS.

In conclusion, adopting a PCOS diet may have various advantages, including managing insulin levels, lowering inflammation, boosting weight reduction, normalizing menstrual cycles, reducing androgen levels, and enhancing fertility. While there is no single "PCOS diet," making small, sustainable changes to your eating habits, such as focusing on whole, nutrient-dense foods, limiting processed foods and refined carbohydrates, and increasing your intake of protein, fiber, and healthy fats, can help manage symptoms and improve overall health. As usual, it is vital to talk with your healthcare physician or a trained dietitian before making any substantial changes to your diet.

## 1.4 Who should follow the PCOS diet

Polycystic Ovary Syndrome (PCOS) is a hormonal condition that affects roughly 10% of women of reproductive age. Women with PCOS may have increased amounts of androgens (male hormones) and insulin, which may produce various symptoms, including irregular menstrual cycles, acne, weight gain, and reproductive issues. Although there is no treatment for PCOS, dietary adjustments may help treat the illness.

The PCOS diet is meant to help manage insulin levels and decrease inflammation. It promotes whole, nutrient-dense diets and minimizes processed and high-sugar foods. Although the PCOS diet may assist everyone wanting to enhance their general health, specific particular categories of individuals may benefit the most from it.

**Women with PCOS:** The PCOS diet is mainly developed to assist women with PCOS in controlling their symptoms. By lowering inflammation and managing insulin levels, the diet may help improve menstrual regularity, minimize acne, and encourage weight reduction.

**Women with insulin resistance:** Insulin resistance is a common disorder in which the body becomes less responsive to insulin, resulting in high blood sugar levels. Women with PCOS commonly develop insulin resistance. However, it may also occur in women without PCOS. The PCOS diet may be suitable for women with insulin resistance since it prioritizes meals that won't boost blood sugar levels and contains items that can assist in improving insulin sensitivity.

**Women who are overweight or obese:** Women with PCOS are at a higher risk of becoming overweight or obese. Reducing weight might be challenging for people with PCOS, but the PCOS diet can successfully support weight reduction by lowering inflammation and increasing insulin sensitivity. Moreover, weight reduction may assist in improving menstruation regularity and boost fertility.

**Women attempting to conceive:** Women with PCOS may have trouble becoming pregnant owing to irregular menstrual cycles and issues with ovulation. The PCOS diet may be helpful for women attempting to conceive since it promotes nutrient-dense meals that can support hormonal balance and reproductive health.

**Women with high levels of inflammation:** Inflammation is a normal reaction of the body to injury or illness, but persistent inflammation may be hazardous to health. Women with PCOS generally have high levels of inflammation, which may lead to the development of insulin resistance and other health concerns. The PCOS diet aims to lower inflammation by emphasizing whole, nutrient-dense foods rich in anti-inflammatory chemicals.

In summary, the PCOS diet may be helpful for women with PCOS, women with insulin resistance, women who are overweight or obese, women attempting to conceive, and women with high levels of inflammation. Nevertheless, it's essential to remember that dietary changes alone may not be adequate to manage PCOS, and women with PCOS should collaborate with a healthcare professional to build a complete treatment plan that may include lifestyle adjustments, medicines, and other treatments as indicated.

# CHAPTER TWO

## 2.0 The Fundamentals of the PCOS Diet

Polycystic Ovary Syndrome (PCOS) is a hormonal condition that affects up to 10% of women of reproductive age. It is characterized by high amounts of androgens (male hormones) in the body, which may produce various symptoms, including irregular periods, weight gain, acne, and excessive hair growth.

Although there is no treatment for PCOS, food and lifestyle adjustments may help control its symptoms. The PCOS diet regulates blood sugar levels, decreases inflammation, and supports healthy weight control.

The fundamentals of the PCOS diet involve the following:

**Consuming a low-glycemic index diet** involves avoiding or restricting high-carbohydrate items that might increase blood sugar levels. Instead, concentrate on meals abundant in fiber, protein, and healthy fats, such as vegetables, fruits, nuts, seeds, and lean meats.

**Controlling portion sizes:** Although consuming a balanced and healthy diet is vital, limiting portions to avoid overeating and weight gain is also necessary.

**Incorporating regular physical activity:** Exercise is a vital element of controlling PCOS, as it helps improve insulin sensitivity, decrease inflammation, and support healthy weight management. Strive for at least 150 minutes of moderate-intensity exercise every week.

**Handling stress:** Persistent stress may increase PCOS symptoms, so it's vital to find strategies to reduce stress, such as meditation, yoga, or other relaxation techniques.

Considering supplements: Certain supplements, such as inositol, omega-3 fatty acids, and vitamin D, may help control PCOS symptoms. But, it's crucial to consult a healthcare practitioner before taking supplements.

By following the essentials of the PCOS diet, women with PCOS may better control their symptoms and enhance their overall health and well-being.

## 2.1 Items to avoid on the PCOS diet

Polycystic ovarian syndrome (PCOS) is a hormonal condition that affects women of reproductive age. One of the primary signs of PCOS is insulin resistance, which may lead to high blood sugar levels, weight gain, and difficulties decreasing weight. Hence, regulating insulin levels with nutrition is crucial to treating PCOS.

Some meals may increase insulin resistance and other symptoms of PCOS. These are some things to avoid on the PCOS diet:

**Sugar**

Regarding sugar and PCOS, we want to keep them apart as much as possible. This is because sugar alters insulin control and induces inflammation.

Sugar/sucrose consists of 50% fructose and 50% glucose.

Fructose is scarcely found in paleolithic diets, so we must be better suited to consume large amounts of it. The excessive fructose intake of typical western diets deteriorates the intestinal barrier and causes endotoxemia. This is where toxins in our gut leak into the bloodstream and cause an inflammatory response.

The liver processes fructose. This is why high consumption has been linked to liver disease and insulin resistance.

This includes candies, sugary drinks, morning cereals, condiments, and sauces.

Nevertheless, although fructose is detrimental to PCOS, easily accessible glucose isn't all that wonderful either. As stated below, the opposite half of a sugar molecule has its challenges.

**Carbs**

Carbohydrate meals may be categorized as "simple" or "complex." Simple carbohydrates contain easily accessible sugars, including sucrose, fructose, and glucose. Complex carbs, by contrast, are the primary building component of starchy meals.

Carbohydrate items are metabolized into glucose. They then enter the circulation to supply the energy required for optimal metabolism. Food's glycemic index (GI) measures the pace at which it causes blood glucose levels to increase. The greater the GI, the higher our reacting insulin levels will be. Humans are well-adapted to ingesting high-fiber, low-GI carbohydrate diets like root vegetables. Yet, the frequent ingestion of high-GI, glucose-rich meals might develop insulin resistance and worsen PCOS.

This includes items like French fries, white rice, spaghetti, and anything heavy in sugar. Baked products and dishes manufactured from white flour are also crucial to avoid.

## Gluten

Adopting a gluten-free diet for PCOS has gained much traction in our community, and for a good reason.

Gluten is a broad word for the numerous proteins in wheat, rye, and barley. Gluten is known to be the trigger for celiac disease. However, a distinct sort of gluten intolerance known as non-celiac gluten sensitivity is of greater significance to women with PCOS.

This makes it obvious when you consider the effect of gluten on the intestines. Numerous studies have indicated that gluten may induce "leaky gut syndrome" in susceptible persons. Experimental findings reveal that gluten increases intestinal permeability in everyone, even if you're generally healthy.

Similarly, with high fructose ingestion, the degeneration of the intestinal wall lining induces inflammation. This happens when toxins travel from our stomach, where they cause minimal damage, to our blood, where they're not intended to be. For women with PCOS, ingesting gluten adds gasoline to the fire of inflammation. This subsequently affects our metabolic health, body weight, skin, hair, mood, and fertility.

Popular gluten-containing foods include spaghetti, bread, breakfast cereals, and other processed meals.

**Dairy**

Like gluten, there's a shortage of scientific evidence associating dairy intake with PCOS. Valid arguments may be made on both sides of this discussion.

In 2020, researchers did literature on the effects of dairy on PCOS. They observed that a favorable impact could not be established. Dairy may be a predictor of insulin resistance. Only yogurt and fermented dairy appear to lessen the chance of acquiring type 2 diabetes.

Past research has produced varied outcomes with respect to dairy's influence on fertility. The most recent study implies that any correlations are likely to be minor.

The difficulty with most dairy-related research is that they're not intended for women with PCOS. As noted in a recent data assessment, "…studies discussing the effects of milk intake in women with

PCOS are few. Therefore, its positive effect may not be clearly established in this group of patients".

This is a case when clinical expertise is essential.

As a health coach, I've noticed that some women with PCOS may handle dairy better than others. My belief, however, is that without having completed an elimination diet first, the dangers of dairy exceed the advantages.

During my 30-Day PCOS Diet Challenge, all participants became gluten and dairy-free. This helps individuals better understand how they react to various items. It's normal for individuals to realize that certain meals no longer agree with them, even if, prior, they believed differently.

These ladies were suffering from undiscovered dairy intolerance. Like non-celiac gluten sensitivity, this dietary intolerance may harm the intestinal wall lining. When this occurs, the body protects itself with an inflammatory reaction, worsening PCOS symptoms.

It's not simply lactose that causes these types of difficulties. The proteins casein and whey may interact with the immune system too. These proteins are found in most dairy products, including cream, yogurt, and cheese. Butter and ghee are the only dairy items allowed for a PCOS diet. They include trace quantities of casein, whey, and lactose since they're essentially a pure source of milk fat.

**Vegetable Oils**

Vegetable oil is a misnomer for commercial seed oils. These processed oils originate from soybeans, maize, rapeseed (canola), cottonseed, and safflower seeds. Most fried dishes and processed foods will utilize one of these oils. Women with PCOS wish to avoid these foods since they increase inflammation.

Industrial seed oils may produce inflammation due to their imbalance of omega fats. Omega-6 fats create pro-inflammatory metabolites, whereas omega-3 fats give birth to anti-inflammatory compounds. A ratio of from 4:1 to 1:1 omega 6:omega three is considered optimum. Nonetheless, the typical Western diet results in a ratio of 20:1 or greater. Industrial seed oil use is frequently the primary driver of this imbalance. This is because they're substantial in omega-6 fats and low in omega-3s.

This is relevant to women with PCOS as an omega fat imbalance has been connected to various associated health problems. This includes depression, cancer, cardiovascular disease, arthritis, and renal illness.

**Processed Foods**

The trouble with processed foods is that they're generally heavy in sugar and carbohydrates. This impairs proper blood sugar management. They also include vegetable oils, dairy, gluten, and food additives. These compounds may induce inflammation.

Fast food is the prototypical processed food. Yet any agricultural product that's been physically, thermally, or chemically handled is technically processed food. It's vital to recognize here that it's all about the elements rather than the definition.
Salted pig rinds, for example, may be deemed "processed." Yet several types solely include hog skins, and sea salt, making them a fantastic snack. Pringles,

by comparison, contains more than 20 ingredients. And most of them are either carbohydrates, vegetable oil, sugar, or additives.
Delicious but also disgusting.

Processed meats should also be analyzed depending on their ingredients. Additive-free sausages are typically good, but avoiding things like ultra-processed hot dogs is preferable.

The essential take-home here is that if anything comes with a nutrition label, it's worth reading it. If you don't like the sight of the components (or you need to know what they are), it's a dish that's best avoided.

**Alcohol**

From a nutritional standpoint, alcohol is one of the most apparent items to avoid. Alcohol is unneeded, and even uncommon drinking has been related to a higher incidence of liver damage in women with PCOS.

Research has demonstrated that this danger affects all PCOS women independent of body weight.

Moderate alcohol use may affect the equilibrium of estrogen to progesterone. It's also related to lower fertility and is dangerous during pregnancy.

At all doses, alcohol lowers sleep quality. It's also known to reduce self-control and increase cravings. It might be a huge concern if you're working hard on your diet or exercise habits.

## The Bottom Line

PCOS is a condition caused by inadequate insulin control and persistent inflammation. These mechanisms are dialed up or down by the foods we eat. Because of this, dietary adjustment is a powerful strategy for lowering the whole gamut of PCOS-related symptoms.

With the correct lifestyle modifications, women suffering from PCOS may regain control of their health and fertility. As well as counting on healthcare experts and fertility specialists, there's a lot we can do to assist ourselves.

The seven most crucial things to avoid with PCOS are sugar, carbohydrates, gluten, dairy, vegetable oils, processed foods, and alcohol. Limiting or obliterating these items is vital to a long-term healthy eating strategy. You should expect to notice significant improvements in your symptoms if you can.

## 2.2 Foods to include in the PCOS diet

The following nutritious meals may minimize inflammation, keep blood sugar levels in line, and help you maintain a healthy weight to lessen the adverse effects of gastrointestinal troubles and other bothersome symptoms of PCOS.

FIBER

"A high-fiber diet provides several advantages to women with PCOS, such as lower insulin levels, and antioxidants which battle to decrease inflammation, and improved gut bacteria," explains Angela Grassi, MS, RD, LDN, founder of

The PCOS Nutrition Center. (Many high-fiber meals include prebiotics, which feed probiotics and assist in sustaining your gut microbiota.)

Examples of high-fiber foods for a PCOS diet include:
Seeds (chia, flax, sunflower seeds) (chia, flax, sunflower seeds)
Legumes (black beans, lentils, chickpeas) (black beans, lentils, chickpeas)
Berries (raspberries, blackberries, blueberries) (raspberries, blackberries, blueberries)
Whole Grains (bulgur, quinoa, brown rice, whole oats) (bulgur, quinoa, brown rice, whole oats)

LEAN PROTEIN

Consuming lean protein (as opposed to meat higher in saturated fat, like red meat and cured meats) may improve weight reduction and keep you filled for longer.

"When it comes to protein sources, I suggest incorporating 2 to 3 meals of fish per week (avoiding fish with high quantities of mercury), chicken (grilled or baked), and plant-based forms of protein," says James Nodler, MD, site director at CCRM Houston.

Examples of foods rich in lean protein for a PCOS diet include:

Fish (salmon, shrimp, tuna, cod) (salmon, shrimp, tuna, cod)
Lean poultry (skinless chicken and turkey) (skinless chicken and turkey)
Plant protein sources (beans, peas, tofu, tempeh) (beans, peas, tofu, tempeh)

ANTIOXIDANT-HEAVY FOODS

"Because women with PCOS have been shown to have low-grade inflammation, elevated inflammatory signals can raise insulin, contributing to worsening of

PCOS symptoms," Grassi says. "The best inflammation-fighting antioxidant-filled foods include fruits, vegetables, whole grains, and unsaturated fats."

Examples of antioxidant-rich foods for a PCOS diet include:

Fruits (strawberries, blueberries, raspberries ) (strawberries, blueberries, raspberries )
Vegetables (spinach, artichokes, kale) (spinach, artichokes, kale)
Whole Grains (whole oats, whole wheat, quinoa, brown rice) (whole oats, whole wheat, quinoa, brown rice)
Unsaturated fats (nuts like pecans, nut butter, olive oil, avocado) (nuts like pecans, nut butter, olive oil, avocado)Similarly, with high fructose ingestion, the degeneration of the intestinal wall-lining induces inflammation. This happens when toxins travel from our stomach, where they cause

minimal damage, to our blood, where they're not intended to be. For women with PCOS, ingesting gluten adds gasoline to the fire of inflammation. This subsequently affects our metabolic health, body weight, skin, hair, mood, and fertility.

Popular gluten-containing foods include spaghetti, bread, breakfast cereals, and other processed meals.

**Dairy**

Like gluten, there's a dearth of scientific evidence associating dairy intake with PCOS. Valid arguments may be made on both sides of this discussion.

In 2020, researchers did a literature of the effects of dairy on PCOS. They observed that a favorable impact could not be established. Dairy may be a predictor of insulin resistance. Only yogurt and fermented dairy appear to lessen the chance of acquiring type 2 diabetes.

Past research has produced varied outcomes concerning dairy's influence on fertility. The most recent study implies that any correlations are likely to be minor.

The difficulty with most dairy-related research is that they're not intended for women with PCOS. As noted in a recent data assessment, "…studies discussing the effects of milk intake in women with PCOS are few. Therefore, its positive effect may not be clearly established in this group of patients".

This is a case when clinical expertise is essential.

As a health coach, I've noticed that some women with PCOS may handle dairy better than others. My belief, however, is that without having completed an elimination diet first, the dangers of dairy exceed the advantages.

During my 30-Day PCOS Diet Challenge, all participants became gluten and dairy-free. This helps individuals better understand how they react to various items. It's normal for individuals to realize that certain meals no longer agree with them, even if, prior, they believed differently. These ladies were suffering from undiscovered dairy intolerance. Like non-celiac gluten sensitivity, this dietary intolerance may harm the intestinal wall lining. When this occurs, the body protects itself with an inflammatory reaction, worsening PCOS symptoms.

It's not simply lactose that causes these types of difficulties. The proteins casein and whey may interact with the immune system too. These proteins are found in most dairy products, including cream, yogurt, and cheese. Butter and ghee are the only dairy items allowed for a PCOS diet. They include trace quantities of casein, whey, and lactose since they're essentially a pure source of milk fat.

## Vegetable oils

Vegetable oil is a misnomer for commercial seed oils. These processed oils originate from soybeans, maize, rapeseed (canola), cottonseed, and safflower seeds. Most fried dishes and processed foods will utilize one of these oils. Women with PCOS wish to avoid these foods since they increase inflammation.

Industrial seed oils may produce inflammation due to their imbalance of omega fats. Omega-6 fats create pro-inflammatory metabolites, whereas omega-3 fats give birth to anti-inflammatory compounds. A ratio of from 4:1 to 1:1 omega 6:omega three is considered optimum. Nonetheless, the typical Western diet results in a ratio of 20:1 or greater. Industrial seed oil use is frequently the primary driver of this imbalance. This is because they're substantial in omega-6 fats and low in omega-3s.

This is relevant to women with PCOS as an omega fat imbalance has been connected to various associated health problems. This includes depression, cancer, cardiovascular disease, arthritis, and renal illness.

## Processed Foods

The trouble with processed foods is that they're generally heavy in sugar and carbohydrates. This impairs proper blood sugar management. They also include vegetable oils, dairy, gluten, and food additives. These compounds may induce inflammation.

Fast food is the prototypical processed food. Yet any agricultural product that's been physically, thermally, or chemically handled is technically processed food. It's vital to recognize here that it's all about the elements rather than the definition.

Salted pig rinds, for example, may be deemed "processed." Yet several types solely include hog skins, and sea salt, making them a fantastic snack. Pringles, by comparison, contains more than 20 ingredients. And most of them are either carbohydrates, vegetable oil, sugar, or additives.
Delicious but also disgusting.

Processed meats should also be analyzed depending on their ingredients. Additive-free sausages are typically good, but avoiding things like ultra-processed hot dogs is preferable.

The essential take-home here is that if anything comes with a nutrition label, it's worth reading it. If you don't like the sight of the components (or you need to know what they are), it's a dish that's best avoided.

**Alcohol**

From a nutritional standpoint, alcohol is one of the most apparent items to avoid. Alcohol is unneeded, and even uncommon drinking has been related to a higher incidence of liver damage in women with PCOS.

Research has demonstrated that this danger affects all PCOS women independent of body weight.

Moderate alcohol use may affect the equilibrium of estrogen to progesterone. It's also related to lower fertility and is dangerous during pregnancy.

At all doses, alcohol lowers sleep quality. It's also known to reduce self-control and increase cravings. It might be a huge concern if you're working hard on your diet or exercise habits.

**Bottom Line**

PCOS is a condition caused by inadequate insulin control and persistent inflammation. These mechanisms are dialed up or down by the foods we eat. Because of this, dietary adjustment is a powerful strategy for lowering the whole gamut of PCOS-related symptoms.

With the correct lifestyle modifications, women suffering from PCOS may regain control of their health and fertility. As well as counting on healthcare experts and fertility specialists, there's a lot we can do to assist ourselves.

The seven most crucial things to avoid with PCOS are sugar, carbohydrates, gluten, dairy, vegetable oils, processed foods, and alcohol. Limiting or eradicating these items is crucial to a long-term healthy eating strategy. You should expect to notice significant improvements in your symptoms if you can.


2.2 Foods to include in the PCOS diet

The following nutritious meals may minimize inflammation, keep blood sugar levels in line, and help you maintain a healthy weight to lessen the adverse effects of gastrointestinal troubles and other bothersome symptoms of PCOS.

FIBER

"A high-fiber diet provides several advantages to women with PCOS, such as lower insulin levels, and antioxidants which battle to decrease inflammation, and improved gut bacteria," explains Angela Grassi, MS, RD, LDN, founder of The PCOS Nutrition Center. (Many high-fiber meals include prebiotics, which feed probiotics and assist in sustaining your gut microbiota.)

Examples of high-fiber foods for a PCOS diet include:
Seeds (chia, flax, sunflower seeds) (chia, flax, sunflower seeds)
Legumes (black beans, lentils, chickpeas) (black beans, lentils, chickpeas)
Berries (raspberries, blackberries, blueberries) (raspberries, blackberries, blueberries)
Whole Grains (bulgur, quinoa, brown rice, whole oats) (bulgur, quinoa, brown rice, whole oats)

LEAN PROTEIN

Consuming lean protein (as opposed to meat higher in saturated fat, like red meat and cured meats) may improve weight reduction and keep you filled for longer. "When it comes to protein sources, I suggest incorporating 2 to 3 meals of fish per week (avoiding fish with high quantities of mercury), chicken (grilled or baked), and plant-based forms of protein," says James Nodler, MD, site director at CCRM Houston.

Examples of foods rich in lean protein for a PCOS diet include:

Fish (salmon, shrimp, tuna, cod) (salmon, shrimp, tuna, cod)
Lean poultry (skinless chicken and turkey) (skinless chicken and turkey)
Plant protein sources (beans, peas, tofu, tempeh) (beans, peas, tofu, tempeh)

## ANTIOXIDANT-HEAVY FOODS

"Because women with PCOS have been shown to have low-grade inflammation, elevated inflammatory signals can raise insulin, contributing to worsening of PCOS symptoms," Grassi says. "The best inflammation-fighting antioxidant-filled foods include fruits, vegetables, whole grains, and unsaturated fats."

Examples of antioxidant-rich foods for a PCOS diet include:

Fruits (strawberries, blueberries, raspberries ) (strawberries, blueberries, raspberries )
Vegetables (spinach, artichokes, kale) (spinach, artichokes, kale)
Whole Grains (whole oats, whole wheat, quinoa, brown rice) (whole oats, whole wheat, quinoa, brown rice)
Unsaturated fats (nuts like pecans, nut butter, olive oil, avocado) (nuts like pecans, nut butter, olive oil, avocado)

## FOODS WITH ORGANIC WHOLE SOY

A new study published in the journal Nutrients reveals that the isoflavones in soy may improve the odds of becoming pregnant. "Organic whole soy has been demonstrated to boost fertility in PCOS women," Dr. Gersh affirms, "But it must be organically grown and not extensively processed," she adds.
Examples of foods containing organic whole soy for a PCOS diet include:
Miso \sEdamame \sTempeh

## FOODS COMPLIANT WITH THE MEDITERRANEAN DIET

Examples of Mediterranean Diet foods for a PCOS diet include:
- All fruits and vegetables
- Seafood (shrimp, salmon tuna, sea bass) (shrimp, salmon, tuna, sea bass)

- Whole Grains (brown rice, quinoa, couscous) (brown rice, quinoa, couscous)
- Healthy Fats (olive oil, simple, unsalted almonds, avocado) (olive oil, plain, unsalted nuts, avocado)

## FOODS COMPLIANT WITH THE DASH DIET

The DASH diet, initially developed for lowering high blood pressure, may also be helpful to people with PCOS in regulating lower levels of insulin. It primarily emphasizes nutritious carbohydrates, such as fruits, vegetables, and whole grains. "Due to the inclusion of fiber, whole grains prevent rises in your blood sugar and insulin levels. People who are insulin sensitive can better control their weight and enjoy a lower risk of diabetes, heart disease, and stroke," Plano explains. "Plus, lower insulin levels are also related to monthly regularity," she adds.

Examples of DASH Diet meals for a PCOS diet include:

- All fruits and vegetables

Whole Grains (brown rice, quinoa, whole wheat) (brown rice, quinoa, whole wheat)

- Poultry and fish (chicken, turkey, salmon) (chicken, turkey, salmon)
- Legumes (peanuts, chickpeas, peas) (peanuts, chickpeas, peas)
- Nuts and seeds (walnuts, pecans, flaxseeds, sunflower seeds.

## 2.3 How to adapt to the PCOS diet

Polycystic ovarian syndrome (PCOS) is a hormonal condition that affects women of reproductive age, typically causing irregular menstrual periods, weight gain, and trouble conceiving. Although there is no treatment for

PCOS, treating symptoms with lifestyle changes, such as dietary alterations, may dramatically improve quality of life.

These are some measures to shift to a PCOS diet:

1. Reduce processed meals and refined sugars.
2. PCOS is commonly accompanied by insulin resistance, indicating that the body has problems utilizing insulin properly. Insulin resistance may lead to excessive blood sugar levels and weight gain, aggravating PCOS symptoms.
3. Avoiding processed meals and refined sugars may assist in regulating insulin levels and

stabilize blood sugar. Examples of processed foods to avoid include white bread, chips, and sugary snacks. Instead, choose healthy meals like whole-grain bread, fruits, and veggies.

4.  Add more high-fiber foods,Fiber is necessary for digestive health and may help manage blood sugar levels. Women with PCOS should strive to ingest at least 25-30 grams of fiber daily. High-fiber foods include fruits, vegetables, whole grains, nuts, and seeds.
5.  Select lean protein sources
6.  Protein is necessary for creating and repairing tissues and helps to maintain blood sugar levels. Lean protein sources like chicken, fish, tofu, and beans are excellent alternatives for a PCOS diet.
7.  Concentrate on healthy fats

8.  Good fats like those found in avocados, almonds, and olive oil may help to decrease inflammation and increase insulin sensitivity. Add these items to your meals in moderation.
9.  Limit dairy and gluten
10. Some women with PCOS may be sensitive to dairy and gluten. Consider limiting or eliminating these foods to see if they improve symptoms.
11. Keep hydrated
12. Consuming adequate water is vital for general health and may help to minimize bloating and improve digestion. Try to drink at least 8-10 glasses of water every day.

**Examples of a PCOS-friendly diet:**

**Breakfast**: Overnight oats with chia seeds, berries, and almond milk.

**Snack:** Carrot sticks with hummus.

**Lunch:** Grilled chicken salad with mixed greens, avocado, and a vinaigrette dressing.

**Snack:** Apple slices with almond butter.

**Dinner:** Baked salmon with roasted vegetables and quinoa.

**Dessert:** Greek yogurt with berries and a drizzle of honey.

In conclusion, transitioning to a PCOS-friendly diet involves making dietary changes that can help to manage insulin levels, regulate blood sugar, and reduce inflammation. It is essential to consult with a healthcare provider or registered dietitian to create a personalized plan that works for you.

## 2.4 Tips for meal planning on the PCOS diet

Adopting a balanced PCOS diet may help control symptoms and improve overall health. Here are some recommendations for meal planning on the PCOS diet:

**Concentrate on complex carbohydrates:** Instead of simple carbs like white bread and sugary snacks, pick complex carbohydrates like whole grains, fruits, and vegetables. These meals will keep you full longer and help manage your blood sugar levels.

**Select lean protein:** Lean protein sources, including chicken, turkey, fish, and lentils, are necessary for a PCOS diet. These meals will help you feel full and deliver crucial nutrients.

**Incorporate healthy fats:** Good fats like those found in nuts, seeds, avocados, and fatty fish may help increase insulin sensitivity and decrease inflammation.

**Avoid processed foods:** Processed foods may be heavy in sugar, harmful fats, and calories. Instead, concentrate on full, nutrient-dense meals.

**Prepare meals ahead of time:** Meal planning may help you make better choices and save time over the week. Prepare meals and snacks ahead of time to ensure you have healthy alternatives accessible.

**Have balanced meals:** Each meal should contain a combination of complex carbs, lean protein, and healthy fats to keep you feeling content and supply critical nutrients.

**Consider working with a licensed dietitian:** A licensed dietician can help you build a tailored meal plan that suits your nutritional requirements and objectives.

Remember to be gentle with yourself and your body when you adjust your diet. Modest, incremental adjustments might be more durable and beneficial in the long term.

# CHAPTER THREE

## 3.0 Breakfast Recipes on the PCOS Diet

Polycystic Ovary Syndrome (PCOS) is a hormonal condition affecting many women, and nutrition may play a significant role in treating symptoms. Here are some breakfast dishes that are PCOS-friendly:

## 3.1 Chia seed pudding:

It is a popular and healthful breakfast or snack that is simple to prepare and can be adjusted to your preference. Here is a simple recipe, preparation instructions, serving ideas, and some toppings to pair with it:

## Recipe:

- 1 cup unsweetened almond milk (or any other milk of your choosing) (or any other milk of your choice)
- 1/4 cup chia seeds
- 1 tbsp honey or stevia (optional) (optional)
- 1 tsp vanilla extract (optional) (optional)

## Instructions:

1.  In a mixing bowl, whisk together the almond milk, chia seeds, honey or stevia, and vanilla extract (if using) until thoroughly blended.
2.  Let the mixture rest for 5 minutes, and then give it another whisk to avoid clumps.
3.  Cover the bowl and chill for at least 2-3 hours or overnight.
4.  After the pudding has thickened and the chia seeds have absorbed

the liquid, stir it and adjust the sweetness to your satisfaction.

**Serving Suggestions:**

- Serve the pudding as is, in a dish or glass.

- Cover the pudding with your favorite fruits, such as sliced bananas, berries, or mangoes.

- Add some crunch by topping the pudding with granola, chopped almonds, or seeds.

- Sprinkle it with honey, maple syrup, or chocolate sauce for a sweeter treat.

- The recipe above yields 2-3 servings, but you can double or treble it to create a more significant amount.

- The pudding may be kept in an airtight jar in the refrigerator for up to 5 days.

Chia seed pudding is an excellent choice for persons with dietary limitations or searching for a healthy breakfast or snack alternative. It is rich in fiber, protein, and omega-3 fatty acids, which may help keep you full and satisfied throughout the day.

## 3.2 Vegetable omelet

This recipe for a basic veggie omelet may be readily tweaked depending on your specific tastes.

**Recipe:**

- Two eggs
- 1/4 cup chopped veggies (e.g., bell peppers, spinach, onions, mushrooms, tomatoes) (e.g., bell

peppers, spinach, onions, mushrooms, tomatoes)
- Salt & pepper, to taste
- 1 tbsp olive oil or butter

**Instructions:**

1.  Break the eggs into a mixing dish and beat them with a fork or whisk until the yolks and whites are thoroughly combined.
2.  Add the chopped veggies to the bowl and stir thoroughly.
3.  Heat the olive oil or butter in a non-stick pan over medium heat.
4.  Pour the egg and vegetable mixture into the pan and let it cook for a few minutes until the bottom is set and the top is still somewhat runny.
5.  Using a spatula, fold one side of the omelet over the other half to produce a semi-circle shape.

6. Sauté for another minute or two until the eggs are completely set and the veggies are cooked.
7. Move the omelet onto a platter and season with salt and pepper to taste.

**Serving Suggestions:**

Serve the omelet as is, or sprinkle with fresh herbs like parsley or chives for added flavor.
Serve the omelet with whole grain bread, roasted potatoes, or a small salad for an entire morning meal.

Put a piece of avocado or a dollop of salsa or sour cream on the omelet for more creaminess and taste.

This recipe produces a single serving, which may easily be doubled or tripled to feed additional people. Omelets are a terrific way to use up any leftover veggies in your fridge, and they can be eaten any time of day, not just for breakfast!

## 3.3 Greek yogurt parfait

Greek yogurt parfait is a nutritious and tasty breakfast or snack choice that is simple to create and customized to your taste preferences. Here's a basic recipe, preparation instructions, serving ideas, and some toppings to pair with it:

**Recipe:**

1. 1 cup plain Greek yogurt
2. 1/2 cup mixed berries (e.g., strawberries, blueberries, raspberries) (e.g., strawberries, blueberries, raspberries)
3. 1/4 cup granola
4. 1 tbsp honey or maple syrup (optional) (optional)

**Instructions:**

1. Layer the Greek yogurt, mixed berries, and granola in a bowl or glass.
2. Drizzle with honey or maple syrup if preferred.
3. Continue the layering technique until you reach the top of the bowl or glass.
4. Top with more berries and granola for added crunch and taste.

**Serving Suggestions:**

1. Utilize any mix of fruits, nuts, and seeds that you prefer to personalize your parfait.

2. Add a spoonful of cocoa powder to the yogurt for a chocolate twist and stir thoroughly.

3.  Add pineapple, mango, and coconut flakes to the mix to create a tropical variation.

4.  Put the parfait in a mason jar and take it on the go for a nutritious breakfast or snack choice.

This recipe produces one serving but may easily be doubled or tripled to feed additional people. Greek yogurt is packed with protein and calcium, while the mixed berries give fiber and antioxidants. Granola gives a crunchy texture and is a source of carbs for energy.

Overall, Greek yogurt parfait is a tasty and nutritious breakfast or snack choice that can be tailored to fit your tastes and preferences.

# 3.4 Sweet potato hash:

Sweet potato hash is a tasty and nutritious breakfast alternative that is simple to create and customized to your taste preferences. Here's a basic recipe, preparation instructions, serving ideas, and some toppings to pair with it:

Recipe:
- One big sweet potato, peeled and chopped
- 1/2 red bell pepper, chopped
- 1/2 yellow onion, chopped
- Two cloves garlic, minced \s 2 tbsp olive oil
- Salt & pepper, to taste

**Instructions:**

1. Heat the olive oil in a large pan over medium-high heat.

2. Add the sweet potato and simmer for 5-7 minutes, stirring regularly, until it begins to brown.

3. Add the red bell pepper, yellow onion, and garlic to the skillet. Sweet potato hash is a tasty and nutritious breakfast alternative that is simple to create and customized to your taste preferences. Here's a basic recipe, preparation instructions, serving ideas, and some toppings to pair with it:

**Recipe:**

- One big sweet potato, peeled and chopped
- 1/2 red bell pepper, diced \s 1/2 yellow onion, diced \s 2 cloves garlic, minced \s 2 tbsp olive oil
- Salt & pepper, to taste

**Instructions:**

1. Heat the olive oil in a large pan over medium-high heat.
2. Add the sweet potato and simmer for 5-7 minutes, stirring regularly, until it begins to brown.
3. Add the red bell pepper, yellow onion, and garlic to the pan and continue cooking for another 5-7 minutes, until the veggies are soft and the sweet potato is thoroughly cooked.
4. Season with salt and pepper to taste.

**Serving Suggestions:**

- Serve the sweet potato hash as is, or top with a fried egg or two for added protein.
- Add some additional flavor with toppings like avocado, cilantro, or spicy sauce.
- Serve the hash with whole-grain bread or

- fresh fruit for a whole morning meal.
- Use the sweet potato hash as a basis for a breakfast tortilla or wrap.

1. This recipe serves around 2-3 servings but may easily be doubled or tripled to feed more people. Sweet potato hash is a rich source of fiber, vitamins, and minerals, and it's a healthier alternative to typical potato hash. Additionally, it's a beautiful and flavorful way to start your day!

2. Overall, sweet potato hash is a tasty and healthy breakfast choice that can be readily adjusted to fit your tastes and preferences.

# 3.5 Almond flour pancakes:

Almond flour pancakes are a tasty and healthful alternative to regular pancakes. They're gluten-free, low-carb, and packed in protein and healthy fats. Here's a basic recipe, preparation instructions, serving ideas, and some toppings to pair with them:

**Recipe:**

- 1 1/2 cups almond flour
- Two eggs
- 1/2 cup almond milk (or any other milk of your choosing) (or any other milk of your choice)
- 1 tbsp honey (optional) (optional)
- 1 tsp baking powder
- 1/4 tsp salt
- 1 tsp vanilla extract

**Instructions:**

1.Mix the almond flour, baking powder, and salt in a large basin.

2. Mix the eggs, almond milk, honey (if using), and vanilla extract in a separate dish.

3. Pour the wet components into the dry ingredients and stir until thoroughly blended.

4. Heat a non-stick pan or griddle over medium heat.

5. Pour batter onto the pan using a 1/4 cup measuring cup.

6. Sauté for 2-3 minutes on each side until golden brown.

Serving Suggestions:

- Serve the pancakes with fresh berries, sliced bananas, or a drizzle of honey or maple syrup.
- Add some additional protein with a dollop of Greek yogurt or a side of turkey bacon.

- Add some cooked spinach, mushrooms, or avocado to make it a savory meal.
- Serve the pancakes with a cup of coffee or tea for a whole morning meal.

This recipe yields around 6-8 pancakes but may easily be doubled or tripled to accommodate additional people. Almond flour pancakes are a terrific source of protein, healthy fats, and fiber, and they're a tasty and fulfilling breakfast alternative.

Overall, almond flour pancakes are a tasty and nutritious alternative to classic pancakes that can be readily adjusted to fit your tastes and preferences.

# CHAPTER FOUR

## 4.0 Snacks and Appetizers on the PCOS Diet

Polycystic Ovary Syndrome (PCOS) is a hormonal condition that affects many women of reproductive age. One of the primary symptoms of PCOS is insulin resistance, which may make it challenging to regulate weight and can lead to excessive blood sugar levels.

A PCOS diet seeks to control insulin levels by limiting the consumption of refined 6. Cover the pan and heat for 10-15 minutes until the chicken is cooked and the veggies are soft.

# 4.1 Homemade Granola Bars

Homemade granola bars are a terrific PCOS-friendly food that is simple to prepare and can be modified to your desire. Here's an easy recipe for homemade granola bars:

**Ingredients:**

- 2 cups old-fashioned rolled oats
- 1/2 cup chopped nuts (such as almonds, walnuts, or pecans) (such as almonds, walnuts, or pecans)
- 1/2 cup seeds (such as pumpkin or sunflower seeds) (such as pumpkin or sunflower seeds)
- 1/2 cup dried fruit (such as raisins or chopped dates) (such as raisins or chopped dates)
- 1/4 cup honey \s 1/4 cup maple syrup
- 1/4 cup almond butter

- 1 tsp vanilla extract
- 1/2 tsp salt

**Instructions:**

1. Preheat the oven to 350°F and line a 9x9-inch baking dish with parchment paper.
2. In a large basin, mix together the oats, chopped nuts, and seeds.
3. Spread the mixture out on a baking sheet and toast in the oven for 10-12 minutes, stirring regularly, until softly golden brown and aromatic.
4. In a small saucepan, boil the honey, maple syrup, almond butter, vanilla extract, and salt over medium heat, stirring frequently, until the mixture is smooth and thoroughly blended.
5. Pour the mixture over the toasted oat mixture and stir until everything is completely covered.
6. Add the dried fruit and mix to blend.

7. Move the mixture to the prepared baking dish and push down hard to form an equal layer.

8. Bake for 20-25 minutes, until the sides are gently browned.

9. Let the granola bars rest in the pan for 10-15 minutes, then transfer to a wire rack to cool fully.

10. After cold, cut the granola bars into bars or squares.

**Serve and Pairings:**

Homemade granola bars may be eaten as a snack on their own or coupled with other PCOS-friendly meals such as Greek yogurt or fresh fruit. These may also be eaten as a pre-workout snack or an on-the-go breakfast. Keep the granola bars in an airtight container at room temperature for up to a week or in the fridge for up to two weeks. Enjoy

## 4.2 Avo-Tuna Salad Lettuce Wraps

Avo-Tuna Salad Lettuce Wraps are a tasty and healthy PCOS-friendly lunch that is simple to cook and can be tailored to your desire. Here's a basic recipe:

**Ingredients:**

- 2 cans of tuna, drained
- 1 avocado, mashed
- 2 tablespoons of chopped red onion
- 2 tablespoons of chopped celery
- 1 tablespoon of chopped cilantro
- 1 tablespoon of lemon juice
- Salt & pepper, to taste
- Romaine lettuce leaves

**Instructions:**

1. In a medium bowl, mix the tuna, mashed avocado, red onion, celery, cilantro, lemon juice, salt, and pepper. Mix thoroughly.
2. Put a tablespoon of the tuna-avocado mixture on each lettuce leaf.
3. Fold the lettuce leaf around the filling, like a burrito or wrap.
4. Serve and enjoy!

**Serve and Pairings:**

These Avo-Tuna Salad Lettuce Wraps are great on their own, but you can also combine them with other PCOS-friendly meals such as fresh fruit or a side salad. To add extra variation, you may also tweak the dish by throwing in other ingredients like chopped tomato or cucumber. These wraps are also fantastic as a convenient and healthy lunch alternative. Refrigerate any leftovers in an airtight jar in the fridge for up to two days.


## 4.3 Baked Sweet Potato Fries

Baked sweet potato fries are a tasty and healthful PCOS-friendly snack or side dish that is simple to prepare and filled with nutrients. Here's a basic recipe:

**Ingredients:**

- 2-3 sweet potatoes
- 1 tablespoon of olive oil
- 1/2 teaspoon of salt
- 1/2 teaspoon of paprika
- 1/4 teaspoon of garlic powder

**Instructions:**

1. Preheat the oven to 425°F.

2. Peel the sweet potatoes and cut them into thin, even-sized fries.

3. In a large bowl, mix the sweet potato fries with the olive oil, salt, paprika, and garlic powder until they are completely coated.

4. Place the sweet potato fries in a single layer on a baking sheet coated with parchment paper.

5. Bake for 20-25 minutes, rotating the fries over halfway through, until they are crispy and gently browned.

6. Serve and enjoy!

**Serve and Pairings:**

Baked sweet potato fries may be served as a nutritious side dish to any meal or as a pleasant snack on their own. They are also a terrific alternative to ordinary french fries. You may mix them with other PCOS-friendly meals such as a salad or grilled chicken for a full dinner. You may also experiment with other sauces and dips to add additional flavor and diversity to the fries. Some wonderful dip possibilities are hummus, Greek yogurt dip, or guacamole. Refrigerate any leftovers in an airtight jar in the fridge for up to three days.

## 4.4 Spiced Roasted Chickpeas

Spiced roasted chickpeas are a nutritious and appetizing snack that you can simply cook at home. Here's a recipe for you to try:

**Ingredients:**

- 2 cans of chickpeas, drained and rinsed
- 2 teaspoons of olive oil
- 1 teaspoon of ground cumin
- 1/2 teaspoon of smoked paprika
- 1/2 teaspoon of garlic powder
- 1/4 teaspoon of cayenne pepper

- 1/2 teaspoon of salt

**Instructions:**

1. Preheat your oven to 400°F (200°C).
2. Rinse and drain the chickpeas, then pat them dry with a clean cloth.
3. In a bowl, mix together the olive oil, cumin, smoked paprika, garlic powder, cayenne pepper, and salt.
4. Add the chickpeas to the bowl and toss until they are coated evenly with the spice mixture.
5. Spread the chickpeas out on a baking sheet lined with parchment paper.
6. Roast the chickpeas in the oven for 20-25 minutes, or until they are crispy and golden brown.
7. Remove the chickpeas from the oven and allow them cool for a few minutes before serving.

Enjoy your spicy roasted chickpeas as a healthy and tasty snack! You may preserve any leftovers in an airtight jar at room temperature for up to a week.

# CHAPTER FIVE

## 5.0 Major Dishes on the PCOS Diet

When it comes to major meals on the PCOS diet, the focus is on lean protein sources such as chicken, turkey, fish, tofu, and lentils. These meals may help balance blood sugar levels, which is crucial for controlling insulin resistance, a typical symptom of PCOS. Moreover, ingesting protein might help you feel filled for longer, minimizing the chance of overeating.

Carbohydrate consumption should also be carefully examined on the PCOS diet, since too many carbs might aggravate insulin resistance. Thus, major meals should feature complex carbs, such as vegetables and whole grains, rather than simple carbohydrates like refined grains and sweets.

It's also crucial to incorporate healthy fats, such as those found in avocado, almonds, and olive oil, in your main meals. These fats may help regulate hormones and enhance general wellness.

In summary, major meals on the PCOS diet should be oriented on lean protein sources, complex carbs, and healthy fats. By adopting this technique, you may control PCOS symptoms and enhance your overall health and wellness.

# 5.1   One-Pot Chicken   and Vegetable Skillet

Here is a recipe for a One-Pot Chicken and Vegetable Skillet:

**Ingredients:**

- 1 pound boneless, skinless chicken breasts, cut into bite-sized pieces
- 2 cups of mixed veggies (such as bell peppers, zucchini, carrots, and broccoli) (such as bell peppers, zucchini, carrots, and broccoli)
- 1 small onion, chopped
- 2 cloves of garlic, minced
- 1 teaspoon dried oregano
- 1 teaspoon paprika
- Salt & pepper, to taste
- 2 tablespoons olive oil

**Instructions:**

1. Heat the olive oil in a large pan over medium-high heat.
2. Add the chicken and heat for 5-6 minutes, or until browned on both sides.

3. Add the onions and garlic to the pan and simmer for 1-2 minutes, or until fragrant.

4. Add the mixed veggies to the skillet and toss to incorporate.

5. Sprinkle the oregano, paprika, salt, and pepper over the pan and toss to cover the veggies and chicken.

6. Cover the pan and heat for 10-15 minutes, or until the chicken is cooked through and the veggies are soft.

**To serve:**

You may serve the One-Pot Chicken and Vegetable Skillet as is or with a side of rice or quinoa. You may also top it with chopped fresh herbs like parsley or cilantro.

**Health benefits:**

This dish provides an excellent mixture of protein from the chicken and fiber and minerals from the mixed veggies. It is also low in carbs and might be a fantastic alternative for individuals on a low-carb or keto diet. The olive oil used for cooking delivers healthful fats and antioxidants. Also, this recipe is simple to personalize using your favorite veggies, making it a flexible and beneficial supper choice.

## 5.2 Spaghetti Squash and Turkey Bolognese

Here's a recipe for Spaghetti Squash and Turkey Bolognese:

**Ingredients:**

- One medium-sized spaghetti squash
- 1 pound ground turkey
- One small onion, chopped

- Two cloves garlic, minced
- One can (28 ounces) (28 ounces) smashed tomatoes
- One tablespoon of tomato paste
- One tablespoon of olive oil
- One teaspoon of dried basil
- One teaspoon of dried oregano
- Salt & pepper, to taste
- Parmesan cheese for serving

**Instructions:**

1. Preheat the oven to 375°F.
2. Cut the spaghetti squash in half lengthwise and remove the seeds and membranes.
3. Drizzle the interior of each half with olive oil and sprinkle with salt and pepper.
4. Put the squash halves cut-side down on a baking sheet and roast for 35-40 minutes, or until the flesh is soft and can be easily penetrated with a fork.

5. While the squash is roasting, heat the olive oil in a large pan over medium-high heat.

6. Add the ground turkey, onion, and garlic to the skillet and heat until the turkey is browned and the onion is soft.

7. Add the crushed tomatoes, tomato paste, basil, oregano, salt, and pepper to the skillet and mix to incorporate.

8. Lower the heat to low and simmer for 20-25 minutes or until the sauce has thickened.

9. Use a fork to scrape the flesh of the spaghetti squash into strands.

10. Split the spaghetti squash amongst serving dishes and top with the turkey bolognese.

11. Serve with grated Parmesan cheese on top.

**Health Benefits:**

This recipe is a healthier version of a famous spaghetti and meat sauce meal since it switches out regular pasta with nutrient-dense spaghetti squash. Spaghetti squash is a low-carb, low-calorie food that is strong in fiber, vitamins, and minerals. Turkey is a leaner protein than beef or pig and is a rich source of vital minerals such as zinc and vitamin B12. Moreover, using crushed tomatoes and tomato paste in the bolognese sauce gives lycopene, an antioxidant associated with a lower risk of cancer and heart disease. Overall, this meal is a tasty and nutritious alternative that is quick to create and may fulfill any pasta appetite.

## 5.3 Sheet Pan Lemon Herb Salmon with Vegetables

**Ingredients:**

- Four salmon fillets
- 1 lb baby potatoes, halved \s 2 bell peppers, chopped \s 1 big red onion,

chopped \s 1 lemon, thinly sliced \s
4 cloves garlic, minced \s 2 tbsp
fresh herbs (such as parsley, thyme,
and rosemary) (such as parsley,
thyme, and rosemary)
- 3 tbsp olive oil
- Salt and pepper to taste

**Instructions:**

1. Preheat the oven to 400°F (200°C).
2. Line a large baking sheet with parchment paper.
3. Whisk together the minced garlic, fresh herbs, and olive oil in a small bowl.
4. Combine the young potatoes, diced bell peppers, and chopped red onion with half of the garlic and herb combination in a large bowl.
5. Distribute the veggies equally on the baking sheet and bake for 15 minutes.
6. Take the baking sheet from the oven and push the veggies to one side.

7. Put the salmon fillets on the opposite side of the baking sheet and brush them with the remaining garlic and herb mixture.

8. Place the lemon slices on top of the salmon fillets.

9. Sprinkle salt and pepper over the whole sheet pan.

10. Return the baking sheet to the oven and bake for 10-15 minutes, or until the salmon is cooked and the veggies are soft.

11. Serve hot and enjoy.

Sheet pan lemon herb salmon and veggies is a delightful and healthy dinner with several health advantages. These are some of the primary benefits of this dish:

1. High in Omega-3 Fatty Acids: Salmon is a good source of omega-3 fatty acids vital for heart health and brain function. Eating salmon consistently may help reduce inflammation, lower blood pressure, and lessen the risk of heart disease.

2. Rich in Protein: Salmon is also high in protein, which is necessary for creating and repairing structures in the body. Protein helps keep you full and pleased, which can benefit weight control.

3. Filled with Vitamins and Minerals: The veggies in this meal contain a range of vitamins and minerals, such as vitamin C, vitamin A, and potassium. These nutrients help sustain a healthy immune system, enhance eyesight, and manage blood pressure.

To serve this meal better, consider the following:

1. Serve with a Side Salad: A simple side salad of mixed greens or arugula with a little vinaigrette may bring some additional freshness and nutrients to this dinner.

2. Add Whole Grains: Serving this recipe with a side of quinoa, brown rice, or whole wheat bread may provide some additional fiber and complex carbs.

3. Utilize Fresh Ingredients: Utilizing fresh, seasonal vegetables and herbs may boost the taste and healthiness of this recipe. Try to pick organic foods wherever feasible to minimize exposure to toxic pesticides and chemicals.

4. Change the Vegetables: You may modify this recipe by using a variety of veggies depending on your tastes and what's in season. Add broccoli, asparagus, or cherry tomatoes for added color and flavor.

Adding a few easy tweaks can convert this already healthy and tasty dish into an even more nutritious and gratifying supper.

## 5.4 Lentil and Vegetable Stir Fry

Here is a recipe for Lentil and Vegetable Stir Fry that is rich in flavor and nutrition:

**Ingredients:**

- 1 cup lentils, washed and drained
- 2 cups water
- 1 tbsp olive oil
- One onion, diced \s 3 cloves garlic, minced \s 1 red bell pepper, chopped \s 1 yellow bell pepper, diced \s 1 zucchini, diced \s 1 cup broccoli florets
- 2 tbsp soy sauce
- 2 tbsp hoisin sauce
- 1 tsp ginger powder
- Salt and pepper to taste
- Cooked brown rice (optional)

**Instructions:**

1. In a medium saucepan, mix the lentils and water. Bring to a boil over high heat, then decrease the heat to medium and simmer for 20-25 minutes or until lentils are cooked.

2. Heat the olive oil in a large pan or wok over medium-high heat while the lentils are cooking. Add the onion, garlic, and sauté for 2-3 minutes, or until the onion is transparent.

3. Add the bell peppers, zucchini, and broccoli to the pan and stir fry for 5-7 minutes, or until veggies are tender-crisp.

4. Mix the soy sauce, hoisin sauce, ginger powder, salt, and pepper in a small bowl.

5. After the lentils are cooked, drain any excess water and return them to the pan with the veggies. Pour the sauce over the lentil and vegetable mixture and stir. Cook for 2-3 minutes or until everything is thoroughly covered.

6. Serve the lentil and vegetable stir fry hot overcooked brown rice if preferred.

Here are some more recommendations to make this meal even more nutritious:

1. Add Additional Vegetables: This dish is a terrific way to use any leftover veggies in the fridge. Add sliced mushrooms,

shredded carrots, or snow peas to the stir fry for more nutrition and taste.

2. Utilize Brown Lentils: Brown lentils are an excellent source of plant-based protein and fiber. They also have a nutty taste that works nicely with the veggies and sauce in this dish.

3. Select Low-Sodium Sauces: Soy sauce and hoisin sauce may be heavy in salt, which can be hazardous to heart health. Seek for low-sodium variations of these sauces or replace a reduced-sodium tamari sauce.

Following these ideas and adding a few simple tweaks, you can produce a tasty and healthy lentil and veggie stir fry that is excellent for a fast and easy midweek supper.

Lentil and vegetable stir fry is a healthy and tasty dish with various health benefits. These are some of the possible health advantages of having lentil and veggie stir fry in your diet:

1. Rich in fiber: Lentils and veggies are high in fiber, which may help enhance digestive health by reducing constipation and keeping you full for longer durations.
2. Excellent source of protein: Lentils are a fantastic source of plant-based protein, making it a perfect meal for vegetarians and vegans. Protein is vital for maintaining and rebuilding bodily tissues.
3. Low in calories: Lentil and vegetable stir fry is low in calories, making it a good alternative for individuals seeking to reduce or maintain a healthy weight.
4. High in nutrients: Lentils and vegetables are rich in critical vitamins and minerals, such as vitamin C, vitamin K, folate, iron, and potassium.
5. May help decrease the risk of chronic illnesses: Lentil and vegetable stir fry include numerous components that may

help lower the risk of chronic diseases such as heart disease, cancer, and diabetes.

Overall, lentil and vegetable stir fry is a healthy and nutritious food that may bring numerous health advantages.

# CHAPTER SIX

## 6.0 Side Dishes on the PCOS Diet

PCOS (Polycystic Ovary Syndrome) is a hormonal condition that affects many women of reproductive age. The PCOS diet seeks to reduce insulin levels and inflammation in the body, which may help relieve symptoms of PCOS, such as irregular periods, acne, and weight gain.

Regarding side dishes on the PCOS diet, it's vital to concentrate on nutrient-dense meals that are low in added sugars and carbs. Here are some ideas:

1. Roasted Vegetables: Roasting veggies like broccoli, cauliflower, Brussels sprouts, and asparagus can add excellent

taste and nutrients to any meal. These veggies are also low in carbs and rich in fiber, which may help manage blood sugar levels.

2. Green Salads: Green salads are an excellent source of fiber and minerals, such as folate and vitamin C. Add healthy fats like avocado or almonds and lean protein like grilled chicken or shrimp to make it a complete meal.

3. Cauliflower Rice: If you're searching for a low-carb alternative to regular rice, consider cauliflower rice. You can create it at home by pounding cauliflower in a food processor or purchasing pre-made frozen cauliflower rice from the grocery store.

4. Sweet Potato Wedges: Sweet potatoes are an excellent source of vitamins A and C and fiber. Cut them into wedges, mix them with olive oil and spices, then bake them in the oven for a tasty and healthy side dish.

5. Zucchini Noodles: Zucchini noodles, or "zoodles," are a terrific alternative to regular pasta. You may create them at home using a spiralizer or purchase pre-made zucchini noodles from the grocery store. They're low in carbs and rich in fiber and may be combined with various sauces and meats.

When picking side dishes for the PCOS diet, concentrate on whole, nutrient-dense foods. These solutions can help you regulate your insulin levels and minimize inflammation, which may help relieve symptoms of PCOS.

## 6.1 Roasted Brussels Sprouts with Balsamic Glaze

Roasted Brussels sprouts with balsamic glaze is a tasty and healthful side dish that's simple to make. Here's how you can create it:

**Ingredients:**

- 1 pound Brussels sprouts, trimmed and halved
- Two tablespoons of olive oil
- Salt and black pepper, to taste
- Two tablespoons of balsamic vinegar
- One tablespoon honey
- One garlic clove, minced

**Instructions:**

1. Preheat your oven to 400°F (200°C).
2. In a mixing basin, toss the halved Brussels sprouts with olive oil, salt, and black pepper until covered.
3. Put the Brussels sprouts on a baking sheet in a single layer, ensuring they aren't crowded. Roast in the oven for 20-25

minutes or until tender and slightly browned.

4. While the Brussels sprouts are roasting, make the balsamic glaze. Mix balsamic vinegar, honey, and chopped garlic in a small saucepan. Bring the mixture to a simmer over medium heat and cook for 2-3 minutes or until the sauce has thickened slightly.

5. When the Brussels sprouts are done, transfer them from the oven to a serving dish. Pour the balsamic glaze over the roasted Brussels sprouts and toss to cover evenly.

6. Serve immediately and enjoy your wonderful roasted Brussels sprouts with balsamic glaze!

Roasted Brussels sprouts with balsamic glaze may be a delightful and healthful addition to your meals. Following are some of the medicinal advantages and probable adverse effects of this dish:

**Medical benefits:**

1. Rich in nutrients: Brussels sprouts are a good source of vitamin C, vitamin K, vitamin A, folate, and fiber.
2. Anti-inflammatory: Brussels sprouts include kaempferol and quercetin, which have anti-inflammatory qualities that may help lower the risk of chronic illnesses, including heart disease and cancer.
3. May assist in digestion: The fiber in Brussels sprouts may improve healthy digestion by reducing constipation and encouraging the development of good gut flora.
4. Low in calories: Brussels sprouts are low in calories and rich in fiber, making them a perfect alternative for weight control.
5. May boost heart health: The high fiber content in Brussels sprouts may help decrease cholesterol levels, which may lessen the risk of heart disease.

**Possible adverse effects:**

1. Gas and bloating: Brussels sprouts contain complex carbohydrates that might be difficult for some individuals to digest, resulting in gas and bloating.
2. May interfere with thyroid function: Brussels sprouts contain goitrogens, chemicals that may interfere with the part of the thyroid gland in certain persons.
3. May interact with blood thinners: Brussels sprouts' high vitamin K content may interact with blood-thinning medications, so people taking these medications should consult their doctor before consuming large amounts of Brussels sprouts.
4. Allergy: Some people may be allergic to Brussels sprouts and experience symptoms like hives, swelling, and difficulty breathing.

Roasted Brussels sprouts with balsamic glaze may be a nutritious and tasty side dish. Still, it is vital to be aware of possible side effects and to take it in moderation if you have any health concerns or allergies.

## 6.2 Garlic and Herb Roasted Cauliflower

Garlic and herb-roasted cauliflower is a tasty and healthy meal with various health advantages. Cauliflower is a member of the cruciferous vegetable family, which also includes broccoli, kale, and cabbage. These veggies are rich in minerals and antioxidants, which may help fight against many ailments.

**Ingredients:**

- One head of cauliflower, chopped into florets
- Three cloves of garlic, minced
- Two teaspoons of olive oil
- One teaspoon of dried thyme
- 1 teaspoon of dried rosemary
- 1/2 teaspoon of salt
- 1/4 teaspoon of black pepper

**Instructions:**

1. Preheat your oven to 425°F (218°C) and line a baking sheet with parchment paper.

2. Combine the cauliflower florets with chopped garlic, olive oil, thyme, rosemary, salt, and black pepper in a mixing dish. Stir well to coat the florets equally with the seasoning.

3. Place the seasoned cauliflower florets in a single layer on the prepared baking sheet.

4. Roast the cauliflower for 25-30 minutes or until they become golden brown and soft when poked with a fork.

5. Remove the roasted cauliflower from the oven and allow it to cool for a few minutes before serving.

6. Serve the garlic and herb-roasted cauliflower as a side dish or add it to salads, bowls, or wraps for additional flavor and nutrients. Enjoy!

**Health advantages of Garlic and Herb Roasted Cauliflower:**

1. High in Vitamins and Minerals: Cauliflower is a rich source of vitamins C, K, and B6, as well as folate and potassium.

2. Antioxidant Properties: Garlic and herbs include antioxidants that help protect against cell damage and inflammation.

3. Digestive Health: Cauliflower is high in fiber, which helps promote healthy digestion and avoid constipation.

4. Immune System Support: Garlic contains immune-boosting effects and may help guard against colds and flu.

Sides to pair with Garlic and Herb Roasted Cauliflower:

**1. Grilled Chicken:** A chicken breast or thigh works beautifully with roasted cauliflower.

**2. Rice or Quinoa:** Serve the roasted cauliflower over a bed of rice or quinoa for a satisfying and healthy dinner.

**3. Grilled Vegetables:** Grilled zucchini, eggplant, or bell peppers make a terrific side meal to match the roasted cauliflower.

**How to Preserve Garlic and Herb Roasted Cauliflower:**

Garlic & Herb Roasted Cauliflower may be refrigerated for up to 4 days. To keep, put the roasted cauliflower in an airtight container and refrigerate. When ready to eat, reheat in the oven or microwave.

You may also freeze Garlic & Herb Roasted Cauliflower for extended storage. To freeze, put the cooled roasted cauliflower in a freezer-safe container and store it for up to 3 months. To reheat, defrost in the refrigerator overnight and then reheat in the oven or microwave.

# 6.3 Baked Sweet Potato Wedges

Baked sweet potato wedges are a tasty and healthful side dish that's simple to create. Here's a basic recipe:

**Ingredients:**

- 2-3 sweet potatoes, cleaned and dried
- Two tablespoons of olive oil
- One teaspoon paprika
- One teaspoon of garlic powder
- One teaspoon salt
- 1/2 teaspoon black pepper

**Instructions:**

1. Preheat your oven to 400°F (200°C).
2. Cut the sweet potatoes into wedges, approximately 1/2 inch thick. Try to make them all a similar size, so they cook evenly.
3. Whisk together the olive oil, paprika, garlic powder, salt, and black pepper in a small bowl.
4. Put the sweet potato wedges onto a large baking sheet and sprinkle with the

seasoned olive oil. Toss the wedges to make sure they are covered evenly.

5. Place the wedges in a single layer on the baking sheet, ensuring they do not touch each other.

6. Bake in the oven for 20-25 minutes or until the sweet potato wedges are soft and gently browned. Turn them over halfway through baking, so they cook evenly on both sides.

7. Serve hot, and enjoy! These wedges are tremendous or served with a dipping sauce, such as sour cream or ranch dressing.

Baked sweet potato wedges not only taste fantastic, but they also provide a lot of health advantages. These are some of the benefits:

**1. High in nutrients:** Sweet potatoes are an excellent source of fiber, vitamins, and minerals such as vitamins A, C, potassium, and manganese.

**2. Antioxidant properties:** The orange flesh of sweet potatoes includes antioxidants, such as beta-carotene, which may help protect against cellular damage.

**3. May aid digestion:** The high fiber level in sweet potatoes might assist in improving digestion and avoiding constipation.

**4. May encourage healthy blood sugar levels:** Sweet potatoes have a lower glycemic index than white potatoes, indicating they can help maintain blood sugar levels consistent.

As for serving options, baked sweet potato wedges may be served as a side dish with various dishes, such as grilled chicken or fish, or a vegetarian dish like roasted vegetables or tofu. They may also be added to salads or eaten as a snack with a dipping sauce.

To preserve leftover sweet potato wedges, put them in an airtight jar in the refrigerator for 3-4 days. To reheat, throw them in the oven at 350°F (180°C) for 10-15 minutes until warm.

## 6.4  Roasted  Root  Vegetables with Rosemary

Roasted root vegetables with rosemary are an excellent and healthful side dish that can be served with various main dishes. Here's an easy recipe for creating this dish:

**Ingredients:**

- Two medium-sized sweet potatoes, peeled and cut into cubes

- Two medium-sized carrots, peeled and cut into rounds
- Two medium-sized parsnips, peeled and cut into cubes
- One medium-sized red onion, peeled and cut into wedges
- Two tablespoons of olive oil
- Two tablespoons fresh rosemary leaves, freshly chopped
- Salt and black pepper, to taste

**Instructions:**

1. Preheat the oven to 400°F (200°C).
2. Add the sweet potatoes, carrots, parsnips, and red onion in a large mixing basin.
3. Pour the olive oil over the veggies and toss to coat evenly.
4. Add the chopped rosemary leaves to the bowl and stir thoroughly.
5. Season with salt and black pepper to taste.

6. Spread the veggies in a single layer on a wide baking sheet.

7. Roast in the oven for 25-30 minutes or until the veggies are soft and golden brown.

8. Serve hot, and enjoy!

**Optional:** If desired, you may add root vegetables like turnips or beets to the mix.

Roasted root vegetables with rosemary are a healthy and tasty recipe that may give various health advantages. These are some of the benefits of this meal, as well as recommendations for sides and preservation:

**Health benefits:**

**High in fiber:** Root vegetables like carrots, parsnips, and sweet potatoes are rich in fiber, which may help support digestive health and avoid constipation.

Filled with vitamins and minerals: Root vegetables are rich in vitamins and minerals, such as vitamin A, vitamin C, potassium, and iron, which help promote immune function, energy generation, and strong bones.

**Antioxidant-rich:** Rosemary contains antioxidants, which help protect cells from damage caused by free radicals and lessen the risk of chronic illnesses.

Low in calories: Roasted root vegetables with rosemary is a low-calorie meal that might be a fantastic alternative for anyone wanting to maintain weight.

**Sides:**

Roasted root veggies with rosemary combine nicely with several sides, such as brown rice, quinoa, or a leafy green salad.

You may add protein, such as grilled chicken or tofu, to make it more full and gratifying.

Add a dollop of plain Greek yogurt or sour cream on top of the roasted veggies for a creamy and tangy variation.

**Preservation:**

Leftover roasted root vegetables with rosemary may be kept in an airtight jar in the refrigerator for up to four days.

You may also freeze the meal for up to three months. To reheat, just set the frozen veggies on a baking sheet and bake them in the oven at 350°F for 15-20 minutes or until cooked.

# CHAPTER SEVEN

# 7.0 Sweets on the PCOS Diet

Regarding sweets on the PCOS diet, there are a few things to remember. First, minimizing sugar consumption and processed carbs is vital since they may increase blood sugar and aggravate insulin resistance. Instead, concentrate on sweets that are lower in sugar and higher in fiber and protein, which may help keep you feeling full and pleased.

These are some examples of PCOS-friendly desserts:

**1. Fresh fruit:** Fresh fruit is a terrific alternative for a sweet treat packed with fiber and minerals. Try chopping up some berries or melon and topping them with a dollop of Greek yogurt for a protein boost.

**2. Chia seed pudding:** Chia seed pudding is a tasty and substantial treat filled with fiber and healthy fats. Just combine chia seeds with almond milk or coconut milk and let it lie in the fridge overnight. Top with fruit or nuts for added taste.

**3. Dark chocolate:** Dark chocolate is lower in sugar than milk chocolate and includes antioxidants that may have health advantages. Go for at least 70% cacao brand and enjoy a little square or two as a treat.

**4. Protein bars**: Seek protein bars that are low in sugar and include at least 10 grams of protein. They may be a handy and enjoyable dessert alternative while you run.

**5. Baked fruit:** Baking fruit may help bring out its natural sweetness without adding sugar. Try baking an apple or pear with cinnamon and a sprinkle of honey for a warm and comfortable dessert.

Remember, eating sweets in moderation is vital, even if they're PCOS-friendly. Adhere to proper portions, and balance your diet with nutrient-rich whole foods.

# 7.1 Chocolate Avocado Pudding

Chocolate Avocado Pudding is a tasty and healthful dessert that's simple to cook at home. Here's a basic recipe to get you started:

**Ingredients:**

- Two ripe avocados
- 1/2 cup cocoa powder
- 1/2 cup maple syrup or honey
- 1/3 cup milk of choice

- 1 tsp vanilla extract \s sprinkle of salt
- Possible toppings: chopped almonds, shredded coconut, fresh fruit, whipped cream

## Instructions:

1. Cut the avocados in half and remove the pits. Scoop out the flesh and throw it in a blender or food processor.
2. Add the cocoa powder, maple syrup or honey, milk, vanilla extract, and salt to the blender or food processor.
3. Mix until smooth and creamy, scraping down the sides as required.
4. Divide the pudding into serving plates or ramekins and refrigerate in the refrigerator for at least 30 minutes.
5. Top with your preferred toppings before serving.

Chocolate Avocado Pudding offers various health advantages owing to its major components - avocados and chocolate powder.

Avocados are an excellent source of healthy fats, fiber, potassium, vitamins, and minerals. They have been associated with many health advantages, such as enhanced heart health, better digestion, and decreased risk of certain illnesses.

On the other hand, Cocoa powder is high in flavonoids, antioxidants that may help protect against oxidative damage in the body. It has been related to various health advantages such as enhanced brain function, decreased blood pressure, and reduced risk of heart disease.

These are some possible health advantages of Chocolate Avocado Pudding:

**1. Increased heart health:** The beneficial fats in avocados and flavonoids in cocoa powder may help enhance heart health by lowering inflammation and improving blood lipid levels.

**2. Better digestion:** The fiber in avocados may help promote improved digestion and reduce constipation.

**3. Decreased inflammation:** The flavonoids in cocoa powder may help reduce inflammation associated with various chronic conditions.

**4. Lowered blood pressure:** The antioxidants in cocoa powder may help decrease blood pressure and enhance overall cardiovascular health.

As for sides, Chocolate Avocado Pudding may be consumed on its own or topped with several toppings such as chopped nuts, shredded coconut, fresh fruit, or whipped cream.

To preserve the pudding, put it in an airtight jar in the refrigerator for 3-4 days. The pudding may thicken in the fridge, so you may whisk in a little additional milk to thin it down if required before serving.

## 7.2 AIP Apple Crisp

Here's a recipe for an AIP (Autoimmune Protocol) Apple Crisp:

**Ingredients:**

- Six medium-sized apples, peeled and sliced
- 1/2 cup coconut flour
- 1/2 cup unsweetened shredded coconut
- 1/2 cup coconut oil, melted
- 1/4 cup honey

- 1 tsp cinnamon
- 1/4 tsp sea salt

**Instructions:**

1. Preheat your oven to 350°F (175°C).
2. Mix the coconut flour, shredded coconut, cinnamon, and sea salt in a bowl.
3. Pour in the melted coconut oil and honey, and whisk until thoroughly incorporated.
4. Mix the sliced apples with some cinnamon in a separate dish.
5. Move the apple slices to a baking dish, and sprinkle the crumble mixture evenly.
6. Bake for 40-45 minutes until the apples are soft and the topping is golden brown.
7. Remove from the oven and cool for a few minutes before serving.
Enjoy your tasty and nutritious AIP Apple Crisp!

**Health Benefits:**

This AIP Apple Crisp recipe is a healthier alternative to traditional apple crisp dishes that generally include refined sugars and flour. This recipe contains gluten-free coconut flour and shredded coconut, which offer dietary fiber, healthy fats, and protein. Apples are also an excellent source of fiber, vitamin C, and antioxidants. Honey is used as a natural sweetener instead of refined sugar. This dish is suited for persons following the Autoimmune Protocol, a nutritional plan that tries to decrease inflammation.

**Sides:**

This AIP Apple Crisp is excellent but may also be served with dairy-free coconut whipped cream or yogurt for added smoothness. For extra crunch, you may also add some chopped nuts, such as pecans or walnuts.

**Preservation:**

This AIP Apple Crisp may be kept in an airtight jar in the refrigerator for up to three days. To reheat, put in the oven at 350°F (175°C) for approximately 10 minutes or until cooked. You may also freeze the apple crisp for up to three months. To reheat, refrigerate in the refrigerator overnight and then reheat in the oven at 350°F (175°C) for approximately 10-15 minutes or until cooked through.

## 7.3   Chocolate   Chia   Seed Pudding

Chocolate chia seed pudding is a tasty, healthful, simple treat. Here's a basic recipe:

**Ingredients:**

- 1/4 cup chia seeds
- 1 cup unsweetened almond milk (or any other milk of your choice)
- 2 tablespoons unsweetened chocolate powder
- 2 tablespoons maple syrup or honey (or any other sweetener of your choice)
- 1/2 teaspoon vanilla extract

**Instructions:**

1. In a mixing bowl, whisk the chia seeds, almond milk, cocoa powder, sweetener, and vanilla extract until thoroughly blended.

2. Cover the bowl and refrigerate for at least 2-3 hours, or overnight, until the pudding has thickened to your preferred consistency.

3. After the pudding is set, give it a thorough stir to break up any clumps and make it smooth.

4. Serve the chilled pudding with fresh berries, chopped almonds, or any other toppings you choose.

Enjoy your healthy and tasty chocolate chia seed pudding!

**Health benefits:**

Chocolate chia seed pudding is a nutritious dessert choice that provides various health advantages, such as:

1. **High in fiber:** Chia seeds are a good source of dietary fiber, which helps regulate digestion and avoid constipation.

2. **Rich in protein:**Chia seeds are also a vital source of protein, which is needed for muscle repair and development.

3. **Filled with antioxidants:** Cocoa powder includes flavonoids, which may

help decrease inflammation and protect against chronic illnesses.

**4. Low in calories:** Chia seed pudding is a low-calorie dessert that may help you fulfill your sweet desire without sacrificing your diet.

**Side effects:**

Although chia seed pudding is typically safe to ingest, it may produce specific adverse effects in some individuals, such as:

**1. Allergies:** Chia seeds are a frequent allergen and may trigger allergic responses in certain people.

**2. Digestive difficulties:** Some individuals may develop digestive issues such as bloating, gas, or diarrhea if they ingest too many chia seeds.

**Preservation:**

Chia seed pudding may be kept in an airtight jar in the refrigerator for up to 5 days. Whisk in additional milk before serving to prevent the pudding from getting too thick. It's also better to keep any toppings separately and add them shortly before serving to avoid them becoming soggy.


## 7.4 Banana Lovely Cream

Banana lovely cream is a healthful and tasty dessert that's simple to create. Here's a basic recipe:

**Ingredients:**

- Two ripe bananas, peeled and frozen
- 1/4 cup of milk of your choice (almond, coconut, etc.) (almond, coconut, etc.)
- 1/2 teaspoon vanilla extract
- Possible toppings: chopped nuts, fresh fruit, chocolate chips, etc.

**Instructions:**

1. Chop the frozen bananas into bits and toss them in a blender or food processor.
2. Add the milk and vanilla essence to the blender or food processor.
3. Mix the ingredients until smooth and creamy, pausing to scrape down the sides as required.
4. If the mixture is too thick, add more milk for consistency.
5. After the excellent cream is smooth and creamy, add it to a bowl and top with your preferred toppings.

6. Serve immediately and enjoy your healthy and tasty banana lovely cream!

**Health benefits:**

Banana lovely cream is a healthier alternative to standard ice cream and has various health advantages, such as:

**1. High in potassium:** Bananas are a rich source of potassium, which may help control blood pressure and avoid heart disease.

**2. Low in calories:** Banana pleasant cream is a low-calorie dessert that may help you fulfill your sweet desire without sacrificing your diet.

**3. Rich in fiber:** Bananas are an excellent source of dietary fiber, which may help regulate digestion and avoid constipation.

**4. Filled with vitamins:** Bananas are an excellent source of various vitamins, including vitamin C, vitamin B6, and folate, which are necessary for general health and wellness.

**Side effects:**

Although lovely banana cream is usually safe to ingest, it may produce specific adverse effects in some individuals, such as:

**1. Allergies:** Some individuals may be sensitive to bananas and develop adverse symptoms such as itching, swelling, or trouble breathing.

**2. Digestive difficulties:** Some individuals may develop digestive issues such as bloating, gas, or diarrhea if they eat too many bananas.

**Preservation:**

Banana lovely cream is best enjoyed shortly after preparing it. But, if you have leftovers, you may keep them in an airtight container in the freezer for up to a week. Before serving, let the fabulous cream melt for a few minutes to soften.

# CHAPTER EIGHT

# 8.0 Suggestions for Sticking to the PCOS Diet

Polycystic Ovary Syndrome (PCOS) is a hormonal condition that affects women of reproductive age. One of the most effective ways to manage PCOS symptoms is through diet and lifestyle modifications. However, sticking to a PCOS diet can be challenging, especially when faced with tempting foods that can aggravate the condition.

In this context, several tips and strategies can help individuals with PCOS stick to their diet and achieve their health goals. These tips include identifying PCOS-friendly foods, planning meals and snacks ahead of time, keeping a food diary, incorporating regular physical activity, managing stress, and seeking support from family, friends, or a healthcare provider.

By applying these techniques, persons with PCOS may make appropriate food choices that can help control their symptoms and enhance their overall health and wellness.

## 8.1 Preparing and Prepping Meals in Advance

One of the essential tactics for keeping to a PCOS diet is planning and cooking meals in advance. This strategy may help persons with PCOS make better choices and avoid temptations that might worsen their illness. Here are some systems for planning and preparing meals in advance:

**1. Establish a weekly food plan:** Make a weekly meal plan that includes breakfast, lunch, supper, and snacks. Be sure to incorporate a range of PCOS-friendly meals, such as lean proteins, complex carbs, healthy fats, and high-fiber foods.

**2. Grocery shop with a list:** After your meal plan, compile a list of the items you need and adhere to when shopping. This might help you avoid impulsive buys and remain on track with your diet.

**3. Prep ingredients:** Spend some time at the beginning of the week to prep items such as cutting vegetables, preparing grains, and marinating meats. This may save time over the week and simplify washing together healthful meals.

**4. Cook in batches:** Make considerable amounts of food, such as soups, stews, and casseroles, that can be portioned up and frozen for later use. This may be a fantastic time-saver and guarantee that you always have healthy alternatives.

**5. Carry snacks and meals:** If you are on the move or have a hectic schedule, prepare nutritious snacks and meals to take with you. This may help you avoid fast food and vending machine items that may need to be PCOS-friendly.

By planning and cooking meals in advance, persons with PCOS may make healthy choices and keep to their nutritional objectives. This can lead to better symptom management and improved overall health and well-being.

## 8.2. Finding Support and Accountability

Finding support and accountability can be crucial for individuals with PCOS trying to stick to a healthy diet. Here are some tips for finding support and accountability:

**1. Join a support group:** Consider joining a support group for women with PCOS. These groups can provide a supportive and understanding community offering advice, motivation, and encouragement.

**2. Work with a healthcare provider:** A healthcare provider, such as a registered dietitian or endocrinologist, can provide guidance and support for individuals with PCOS. They can help create a personalized nutrition plan, monitor progress, and adjust as needed.

**3. Enlist a friend or family member:** Share your goals and struggles with someone who can provide accountability and support. They can help keep you on track and celebrate your successes.

**4. Utilize social media:** Social media may be a tremendous source of support and encouragement. Try following accounts that concentrate on PCOS-friendly meals, exercise, and lifestyle suggestions.

**5. Monitor progress:** Keep track of your progress using a food journal or a tracking app. This might help you keep responsible and make modifications as required.

By finding support and accountability, individuals with PCOS can feel more confident and motivated to stick to a healthy diet. This may lead to better symptom management and increased overall health and well-being.

## 8.3 Managing Cravings and Temptations

Managing cravings and temptations can be challenging when sticking to a PCOS diet. Here are some tips to help manage cravings and resist temptations:

**1. Identify trigger foods:** Identify the foods that trigger your cravings and temptations. These may include sugary foods, processed foods, and high-fat foods. Once you have identified your trigger foods, limit or avoid them as much as possible.

**2. Plan for treats:** Allow yourself the occasional treat or indulgence. Prepare for it in advance and enjoy it in moderation. This may help minimize feelings of deprivation and lessen the probability of overeating harmful foods.

**3. Have healthy snacks:** Keep nutritious snacks on hand to fulfill cravings and avoid hunger. Excellent alternatives include fresh fruit, nuts, seeds, and vegetables with hummus or yogurt dip.

**4. Keep hydrated:** Drink lots of water throughout the day. Occasionally, thirst may be mistaken for hunger, and keeping hydrated can help lessen cravings and temptations.

**5. Perform stress-reducing activities:** Practice stress-reducing activities such as yoga, meditation, or deep breathing techniques. Stress may increase desires and temptations; therefore, reducing stress can be helpful.

**6. Get enough sleep:** Obtain proper sleep each night. Lack of sleep may boost hunger and the desire for unhealthy meals.

Using these guidelines, persons with PCOS may control their desires and temptations and maintain a balanced diet. This may lead to better symptom management and increased overall health and well-being.

## 8.4. Remaining Inspired and Focused on Your Health Objectives.

Remaining motivated and focused on health objectives may be challenging, particularly when facing setbacks or hurdles. Here are some ways to help keep motivated and focused on your PCOS health goals:

**1. Establish reasonable objectives:** Create realistic goals that are feasible and quantifiable. Divide huge objectives into smaller, more attainable ones, and celebrate each success.

**2. Build a vision board:** Make a vision board that depicts your objectives and inspires you to remain on track. Include pictures, quotes, and affirmations that encourage and remind you of your vision.

**3. Celebrate progress:** Celebrate your progress and accomplishments, no matter how small. Acknowledge your efforts and give yourself credit for your steps towards better health.

**4. Surround yourself with positivity:** Surround yourself with positive people and environments that support your goals. Avoid negativity and people who may discourage you from pursuing your health goals.

**5. Stay informed:** Stay informed about PCOS and its management. Learn about the benefits of a healthy diet and lifestyle and how they can improve your symptoms and overall health.

**6. Practice self-care:** Practice self-care regularly, and make time for enjoyable activities. This can help reduce stress and improve your overall well-being.

**7. Seek support:** Seek support from family, friends, or healthcare providers who understand and support your goals. They can provide encouragement and motivation when you need them most.

By utilizing these techniques, persons with PCOS may remain motivated and focused on their health objectives, even when facing hurdles or setbacks. This may lead to better symptom management and increased overall health and well-being.